THE REAL
PERFECT 10

THE REAL
PERFECT 10

10 RULES TO SAVE THE HEALTH OF AMERICAN GIRLS (AND EVERYONE ELSE)

ASHLEY NICOLE KORFF

authorHOUSE®

AuthorHouse™
1663 Liberty Drive
Bloomington, IN 47403
www.authorhouse.com
Phone: 1-800-839-8640

Published by AuthorHouse   06/13/2012

ISBN: 978-1-4772-1035-2 (sc)
ISBN: 978-1-4772-1033-8 (hc)
ISBN: 978-1-4772-1034-5 (e)

Library of Congress Control Number: 2012909493

Any people depicted in stock imagery provided by Thinkstock are models, and such images are being used for illustrative purposes only.
Certain stock imagery © Thinkstock.

This book is printed on acid-free paper.

DEDICATION

To anyone who has struggled with weight ...
gone through what I have . . . been teased,
ridiculed, bullied because of being the
fat kid . . . humiliated and embarrassed
because of being fat . . . I'm here to say
being fat wasn't easy, but what I've done
and accomplished, the sweat and heart
and soul I put into changing not just my
weight but my life-that's the greatest feeling
ever to be felt. It's an emotional high that
no one else on earth could ever give you
because it all depends and thrives on the
hard work physically and mentally you put
in. No matter how hard the going gets, don't
give up. This extremely healthy lifestyle I
live and this book are for you, the faces of
obesity and the hearts of determination and
accomplishment.

CONTENTS

Everything you're doing and think of nobody but you now! YOU have opened this book and you are going to FINISH it and CHANGE your life-you only get ONE LIFE so make it the BEST POSSIBLE!

PART 1

THE RULES

1. Motivate Yourself!

You can only turn to yourself for motivation. Nobody else puts food in your mouth, pushes PLAY on your DVD player, or ties up your workout shoes . . . so why count on anybody else for willpower? Willpower comes to the mind on its own but can also be tattooed there from extreme determination. There is no other mind like a human's . . . willpower is something that can turn your life from ordinary into extraordinary. Every time someone hurts your feelings, brings you down, makes you mad, teases you because you're overweight, IGNITE that anger and helplessness into a freaking WILDFIRE, baby!! Show them who's boss!! So who's in control of your life and motivation? YOU are! Find what motivates you. It may be different from someone else's, but that's the whole point! No one body or mind is universal. What motivated me as an overweight middle school kid was the years and years of wanting to wear the same clothes the thin girls got to wear and the humiliation of feeling like the clumsy fat kid all the time. I remember looking in dressing room mirrors and wondering why I could not look like all the other girls at school. I was always the kid that had issues in gym class and had to change in the showers out of sheer embarrassment. I was fed up with being the outsider kid, the fat girl, the one people were nice to because they didn't know otherwise. Every time I felt like not doing a workout, any day when I felt like crap from a headache or something, those were the days I was glad I didn't skip a workout. I pulled out the dark memories of humiliation and embarrassment and used that as fuel to the workout fire. No one else will ever give you the motivation that's innate, or within yourself. I know that sounds far-fetched at first, but trust me on this. Don't let a sick kind of day or lazy day damper your motivation, no matter how hard the going gets. Digging deeper and blasting out all that anger and depression and any other emotion in a workout is the best medicine in the world. And by having all that built-up motivation at the ready, you'll be burning calories and getting in shape while pretending to beat the living crap out of someone that made you mad in a kickboxing class. Motivation is the ultimate win-win situation.

2. Do Workouts You Enjoy

If you don't enjoy a certain kind of workout, you and I both know you won't do it. Just because a lot of people like a workout, whether it's a machine at the gym or workout tapes, does not mean everyone will love it. If running on a treadmill spells death and disaster for you, don't run on a treadmill! Simple as that! Find something else you enjoy doing-cycling, swimming, kickboxing (my personal fav), walking! Any and all kind of exercise is great for you and will turn you into a fat burning machine if you stick with it! But you can't stick with the program if you dread it, right? Forget the hype and remember which workouts you love-and do those workouts! You have to do workouts you love to get a body you love! Also, pushing yourself has to be a major factor. Don't just do a workout because you know it's easy; instead, improve by going harder, farther, and faster in the workouts you love. Now, the low-down on the sweat for those workouts: some people sweat more than others, no matter how hard they push in a workout or race. It's all got to do with genetics and the environment you're working out in. So if you're not dripping buckets of sweat by the end of a favorite workout, don't think you didn't get a decent workout in. As long as you push yourself throughout a workout, you gave your best, so forget about the sweat. Hotter conditions and cardio will usually make me sweat more than colder conditions and resistance training. By doing workouts you love (or at least like), you'll be more likely to push yourself, so chances are you better have water and a towel to handle the sweat, especially if you're a heavy-sweater. Ho-hum workouts usually are completed on autopilot with total disinterest (I can definitely vouch for the several tapes and routines I found boring). Awesome workouts will make you enjoy working out, encourage you to go the extra mile, and maybe even make a light-sweater sweat buckets!

3. No Diet Is One Fits All

You cannot escape the diet fads out there because they are everywhere, from high protein to low fat to low carb to extremely low calorie. So which one is the best? That answer depends on every individual person. You won't believe how many people have tried a promised fad diet and have not succeeded. Why? Because everyone's metabolism runs differently . . . no two bodies are 100% exactly alike. Therefore, no two metabolisms run the same way. You could have a relative that gets great results with a low fat diet, but you could find you need a high protein diet.

The key is to pick healthy foods and you will achieve great results. When following a certain kind of diet, don't get disappointed if it doesn't work the way you wanted. I used to scan magazines that claimed the "healthiest" foods and such and take them to heart. I realized that even though all foods claimed to be "healthy" aren't made equal, wasting the time and energy to craft the upmost ideal diet plan isn't worth it because it doesn't exist. Each body is physically different chemically from others, so that means certain food and portions could be registered differently. Generally, the best health diet is just avoiding high fat and sugar food because fat and sugar is what packs on the pounds. Once I cut fatty and sugary food out, the pounds melted off-something that all those magazines and fad diets can't vouch for.

4. THE DISH ON HEALTHY FOOD

Avoid white carbs, sweets, junk food, and higher fat meat (pork, sausage, pepperoni, etc.) and you have yourself a healthy diet. People often get too caught up on the "organic" and "overprocessed" foods, and there's nothing wrong with that. But trying to buy everything organic can turn into a nightmare both mentally and financially. So eat fruits, veggies, low fat or fat free dairy, lean meat, and wheat and whole grain carbs, and you will be good to go. CHILL out with the labels . . . don't even go down the junk food aisle! You can spend your time overanalyzing which fruits melt fat the fastest or you could be spending your time having fun. ALL healthy foods are equally healthy. Yes, different healthy foods have different vitamins and nutrients, but that doesn't make one better than another. Eat which healthy foods you like, and just forget about the ones that make you want to vomit. Don't like raw veggies? Steam or bake them, and forget about "raw veggies have the most nutrients" gig. If you don't eat raw veggies, you won't get any health benefits from it because you are not eating veggies.

5. BEWARE OF LATE-NIGHT SNACKS (AND MEALS!)

Eating late at night is a HUGE pitfall for a lot of people, since adolescents and adults tend to stay up really late into the night. And when you stay up late, your stomach does, too. And then it starts to growl, so you grab whatever snack or meal you want since you're still awake. Sounds reasonable, right? WRONG! Those extra calories are most likely not being put to good use-watching TV, being on the computer, and/or cramming for a test does not count as physical activity.

But then why does your stomach want food? Your body fasts naturally overnight, but you don't react until breakfast time because you're asleep. Unless you're dying of starvation, your body most likely will stay asleep and wait until breakfast to eat. And if you do find you're extremely hungry towards bedtime, eat a little earlier in the day, since this is a signal you're not eating enough in the daytime. Finish all meals and snacks at least an hour and a half before bed so they have time to digest and begun to be burned off. Chowing down on chips, candy, and/or other notorious late night foods adds up to extra pounds. Skip the extra load by adjusting your schedule to an earlier bedtime. Your brain will also thank you by getting much needed sleep! Staying up super late all the time takes a toll on your brain as well as your overall health. You will do yourself a HUGE favor by getting rest and forgoing to the late munchies! And if for some reason you do find yourself up all night (life happens, people), snack on something healthy, like veggies or fruit, if you're feeling famished.

6. BACK AWAY FROM THE SODA AND JUICE AND NO BODY WILL BE HURT!

No, seriously. If you stay away (and you WILL) from soda and juice, you will have a HUGE improvement in your body and overall health. Soda is called diabetes in a can (or also liquid diabetes) for a reason! Soda is nothing but non-nutritional crap that bloats you up and adds flubber to yourself. I could write a book on just this tip in itself-don't get me started on how horrible this is for your body! Diet soda is just as bad (or even worse) than regular soda-don't let the "zero calories" ploy trick you! Sugary drinks are the equivalent of dumping a bag of pure sugar in some water and guzzling it down. Sugary juices are just as bad, too. They have just as much sugar as soda and usually have little or no real fruit juice, despite the rigorous claims presented in ads. Few juice drinks have no added sugar and real fruit juice. When in doubt, leave it out (of your diet and shopping cart)! Can't resist soda and juice still? Imagine the drink as solid and liquid yellow, cheesy fat oozing out of the can, but wait, it gets stuck so it kind of just gloops out of the can like tar. It plops with a plunk into your glass or into your mouth-that decadent, scrumptious glob of yellow, spoiled cheesy goo just looks delicious now, doesn't it? I sure hope not. In all seriousness, people, don't drink sugary drinks. It's that simple-yet for many is always so hard. Just think of the wonderful example I gave of what REALLY goes into your body when you drink a can of soda or juice. Chances are, you won't think twice of heaving all sugary drinks in your house into the garbage.

7. Know What You're Up Against

Whether you have ten or one hundred and ten pounds to lose to get to your happy weight, you MUST know what you will be facing! This is VITAL! If you are premeditated to a thyroid disease that is causing your weight gain or other genetic factors, this information is CRUCIAL to reaching your goal. Genetic factors are out there, so if your doctor has told you that you have one, this could result in a more difficult, but not impossible, weight reduction. Even if your goal is to lose a smaller amount of weight, or even just to improve yourself, KNOW

WHAT YOU WANT. If you don't know what you want or additional factors besides extra weight, your goals become ambiguous. It's like going into a gun fight with a knife. GET your weapon, whether it be extra help with a genetic disorder or just writing down what you want, and GO FOR IT, BABY! You GOT to have a plan to get to the finish line.

8. Stay On Task

Staying on task is the best advice I could give you for anything in life. If you veer too much off course, chances are that you will most likely go farther and farther away from your goals. You not only have to know what you want, you have to STICK with the program, people! What would be the point in wanting and craving the life you want to lead, only to let the entire plan go down the drain?! There would be no point, aside from wasting time. There is no time to waste! You don't let anything else important in your life go to waste because of getting off track, so don't let your health be the first. Just think that when it's over, you will be beyond happy and estatic that you stayed on task and got to where you're going-you will be ignited! If you have never stuck with something in your entire life before, well, this is one of the best things to stick with. You will never, EVER regret staying on task living a healthy lifestyle. Trust me. If a 14-year-old girl can do it, ANYONE can do it. Period. And I have yet to regret it. I will never see that day come-and neither will you.

9. BEWARE LATE-NIGHT SNACKS

This was a huge obstacle for me-forgoing a snack after dinner, right before going to bed. What happened was that the extra food turned into fat stores because it was not being used up. It's really hard at first, I'm not going to lie about that. You get hungry because you're used to eating that extra something. So if you do get hunger pains, eat a healthy snack like raw veggies, and make sure you finish it at least two hours before going to bed. But it's not really that bad anyways, so just skip it. Ice cream and huge bowls of yogurt and cereal were my right before bed downfalls. Media can impact your late-night cravings tremendously, from watching late television shows to seeing ads for fast food joints open until the early morning. The best way to avoid extra junk you don't need, avoid the triggers as much as possible. Flip the channel when a fast food commercial comes on. Go to bed earlier. Avoid going to a midnight movie premiere because where there's movies, there's that buttery tub of popcorn going down your hatch at one in the morning-a classic example that spells DISASTER. Avoiding situations like these will help you out in the short term and in the long run, spelling SUCCESS. The back-up plan: if it's a late-night event that's important or nonnegotiable to you, then lessen your calories during the daytime so you don't overeat, and pick healthy options or just pack your own munchies and bring them to the party or theater.

10. PLAN AHEAD

Getting a routine down is vital to anything in life you want to achieve. If you have a demanding career, school schedule, or just have a busy life, planning workouts and meals ahead of time will do you a world of good. Picking out a time that you know you can stick with a daily workout is crucial. Leaving your workouts to chance means you probably won't find the time to get a workout in. Know whether you like to workout early, during the day, or even in the late afternoon, and stick with it, adjusting to your schedule to make sure you can get a full workout in. Letting your meals and snacks up in the air on a busy day can mean turning to bad options for a quick meal. Fast food joints are starting to have healthy options like salads or even yogurt and fruit, so check some places out for calorie count and fat amounts before going in head on without a clue if it really is a good option. Some salad dressings can clock in a huge calorie and fat amount, so get smart about fast food and restaurant options when you're on the fly ahead of time. When in doubt, leave it out! Your first option should be to plan or cook ahead a healthy meal, but life does get in the way. Many restaurants have healthy options on the menu, but use your good judgement. If you know you will go for an old junk food favorite at a restaurant or fast food joint, avoid the place if you don't have the willpower to order something healthy. Yes, that's easier said than done for many people. With time, though, you'll find eating healthier when you're out and about will get easier, especially if you start right from the get go. Getting a weekly routine down pat with planning ahead on really busy days will really get and keep you on track.

PART 2

THE FOOD

YOUR MENU

Watch how easy picking out healthy food is-forget about those complicated and twisted studies and fad diets and blah, blah, blah . . . THIS is pretty much the gist of ALL you need to know about healthy food. READY? (Drum roll please) And here it is . . .

1. Any and ALL fruits and veggies
2. Lean/extra lean meat
3. Nuts and beans
4. Low-fat/fat-free dairy
5. Multigrain/wheat carbs
6. Lowest-fat possible nutrition bars/ powders

Yep, that's it. Pretty awesome, huh? And you were worrying and over analyzing whether blueberries or strawberries were better or if chicken outdoes fish in the meat department. Give me a break! If you only eat the six food groups I just showed you, you will be all good! Stop worrying and stressing out over walnuts being better than peanuts or something irrelevant like that. START worrying about what junk food and soda will do to you if you eat it. START worrying about getting workouts in and doing extra the next time if you skip one. Don't just worry about it, DO something about it! Now, how to cook the healthy food is simpler. Don't believe me? Watch . . .

1. Steam, stir-fry (lemon juice or olive oil only), bake, or broil (SSBB)

When in doubt about how a food is prepared, ask or just leave it out. Cook all your food

SSBB to spell SUCCESS. Ditch frying and using butter to cook with (substitute butter with applesauce or yogurt in baked goods), white flour (use wheat flour instead), and a ton of sugar (use yogurt or just leave it out) to see a major improvement in your body and health.

Now here's some lovely recipes to get you started . . .

MAIN DISHES

Teriyaki Salmon

-one or several pieces of salmon (depending if you want a one—or multi-person meal)

—2 tbsp teriyaki sauce per salmon filet

—any fish spice if you wish (to taste)

—cooking spray (nonstick)

—lemon juice or water (to coat the bottom of pan)

Preheat the oven to 350 or 425 degrees Fahrenheit (depending on how fast you want the salmon to cook). Spray the bottom of the cooking pan with the cooking spray and drip just a little lemon juice or water to prevent the salmon from burning (this replaces the common favorite butter). Put the salmon in the pan and then coat the filets with the teriyaki sauce and spice. Place the pan in the oven and let the salmon cook for 20-30 minutes until it's done. Test the fish before pulling it out of the oven to make sure it's done well to prevent food poisoning-better safe than sorry!

Healthy Chinese Stir-Fry

—one or more chicken breasts (fat removed; number of breasts depends on individual or family meal)

—as much broccoli, carrots, water chestnuts, mushrooms, bell pepper, and onion you want in your dish

—one-half or two cans mandarin oranges and/or pineapple (single or multi-person meal), with juice completely drained (or ½—2 cups fresh)

—2 tbsp teriyaki sauce per chicken breast

—ginger and garlic salt (or other Asian spice mixes) to taste

—nonstick cooking spray

—1/2 cup lemon juice

—1 cup water (to prevent burning; add more if needed, especially for a multi-person meal)

Prepare chicken breasts and cut the fat off. Spray the wok or pan with the cooking spray thoroughly and add the lemon juice. Cook the chicken while chopping the veggies into bite-sized pieces or chunks. Stir the chicken when needed and cook until it's well done. Remove chicken (keep in a covered dish) to cook the veggies, adding water when needed so the veggies won't burn. Add the chicken into the wok with the veggies and then add the teriyaki sauce and spice, mixing it all so the sauce gets on everything. Add the mandarin oranges and/or the pineapple once everything else is completely done, letting the fruit get warmed through a little. Or you could grill the fruit beforehand if you have more time, but the dish tastes great as it is, too.

MACARONI-AND-CHEESE MAKEOVER!

—any amount of whole wheat macaroni noodles

—as much fat-free shredded cheddar cheese as needed

—rosemary or another herb (if you want)

—whole-wheat bread crumbs (if you bake the macaroni with a crust)

—nonstick cooking spray (if baking)

Fill a pot with water and set the stovetop setting on high. Add the noodles when the water's boiling. If you're baking the macaroni and cheese and you want a crust, use a baking pan and spray it with the nonstick cooking spray. Preheat the oven to 350 degrees Fahrenheit and grab the wheat bread crumbs. You can make your own by toasting wheat bread and crumbling the finished toast. Take the noodles off the stovetop once they're done and drain out the water. Put the noodles in a bowl or the pan if you're baking. Mix in the fat-free shredded cheddar cheese until melted. Just put the cheese and crumbs on top of the noodles in the pan if you're baking it, then put it in the oven for 5 minutes to heat it through.

DESSERTS

Any of these quick and healthy dessert options will have you stop eating fattening desserts from the restaurant, freezer section, and even your own kitchen! These are all delicious, trust me-I used to chow down on my fair share of unhealthy junk desserts until I found out these very healthy and super-yummy alternatives!

1. Fruit, yogurt, and/or protein powder smoothie: Add any combination of fruit, yogurt, and protein powder you like to a blender and mix!

2. Chocolate pudding: Mix chocolate protein powder in vanilla yogurt

3. Peppermint mocha: Stir a spoonful of chocolate protein powder in hot water or fat-free milk and add a peppermint (top with fat-free whipped cream if you want)

4. Oatmeal raisin cookies made with whole-wheat flour and applesauce or vanilla yogurt (no white flour or butter/sugar!)

5. Fat-free and/or no-sugar-added frozen yogurt (or just freeze any favorite yogurt cup of yours for a couple hours)

6. Any combination of fresh fruit

7. No Pudge Fudge (sold in various grocery chains): An all-natural, fat-free alternative to the old fattening favorite! Made with wheat flour and prepared with only fat-free vanilla yogurt!

8. Chocolate granola or protein bar

Just by following the cooking guidelines above can make any dish into a healthy remix. No dish is "off limits" if you can make it healthy! What about party foods like pizza and ice cream? Use wheat crust and fat-free cheese and turkey or shrimp on the pizza and buy frozen yogurt instead of ice cream (it tastes the same)! And the cake? Make your own with wheat flour and yogurt instead of butter and sugar (or use a no-calorie sugar substitute) and chocolate protein powder or unsweetened cocoa powder instead of chocolate. Use your creativity to transform comfort food dishes into totally healthy (and still yummy) meals!

Once you get the hang of it, it comes naturally to you. By simply buying the healthier substitutes of everyday baking and cooking goods helps your health a ton. Need some help? There are so many healthy cookbooks and magazines out there to get you started. Get smart about cravings.

That means knowing when and where you get that hankering for something sweet, chocolate, or salty. If you know you're going to be magnetized to the buttery popcorn at the movies every time you go, does that mean you can never go to the movies? Heck, no! Just bring some non-buttery popcorn or another healthy snack in your purse and grab a water bottle. Steering completely clear of the snack bar will help you stay on track. Eat a chocolate-flavored granola bar or have a scoop of chocolate protein powder. Crunch on raw carrots, not those horrific potato chips. Taking those little steps is what is going to spell success for you in the long run.

A Day in My Diet:
Then versus Now

THEN (before losing weight)

Breakfast: sugary cereal or pancakes with syrup and bacon

Snack: something in the sugar or junk department (cookies and snack packs were all-time favorites)

Lunch: Pasta, pizza, or the like with ice cream if at home; pasta, sugary and junk foods (chips, cookies, etc.)

Snack: C-o-o-k-i-e-s (or some kind of seasonal, sugary junk food like candy)

Dinner: Pasta or sometimes seafood (with pasta salad or macaroni and cheese), little to no veggies, baked potato if no pasta at restaurant; three to four large glasses of milk mixed with strawberry sugary drink mix to make strawberry milk; dessert of ice cream or cake/ before bed snack of bowl of ice cream, cereal, or lots of full-calorie yogurt mixed with chocolate mix

Drinks: sugary milk (never plain), juice, soda, maybe water, sports drinks

Daily exercise: no routine whatsoever, recreational sports when in season for one or two days a week for about an hour

Notes: If there were any signs of a holiday or sweets in my vicinity, I would definitely chow down on any holiday candy, cookies, pies, or cakes without hesitation, even right before bed. Eating big bowls of ice cream became a daily basis in the summer. Fast food and pizza became regular several days of the week.

NOW (DURING AND AFTER LOSING 50 POUNDS)

Breakfast: a healthy cereal with fat-free yogurt

Lunch: Protein shake or smoothie with fruit

Snack: Bowl of fresh and dried no-sugar-added fruit

Dinner: Lean meat or seafood with lots of veggies and a salad with fat-free dressing

Drinks: Water, water, and water! Herb tea in the winter (NO SUGAR); no calorie and sugar free flavored water on occasion in the summer

Dessert: A healthy remake (fat-free yogurt used instead of butter and sugar, wheat flour instead of white, etc.) of a dessert or fruit on occasion

Daily Exercise: Two hours a day, every day; I mix up cardio and strength training routines every month or two to change things up.

Notes: I usually alternate my breakfasts, lunches, and snacks every several months or so. When I get hooked on a favorite breakfast or lunch, though, I'll eat it every day for several months. Most people probably want more variety in their meals, though, and that's ok as long as the food is healthy.

PART 3

THE
EMOTIONAL HELP

Nothing frustrates me more than the lack of empathy out there for girls struggling with their weight. All the magazines and media bombard girls of all ages and all backgrounds everyday with the "perfect" image of a girl. I cannot tell you how much it bothered me as a little kid and even today as an older teenager. I used to look at myself and wonder why the heck can't I look like the pretty girls in the movies? I would think about it a lot and hide what I thought of myself: a fat, ugly, clumsy blob.

I'm here to tell you, girls (and guys,too),that I completely empathize with you on your battle with yourself. I have yet to find someone that KNOWS how it feels to be humiliated and embarrassed of yourself. Nobody in my family could understand the mental battle you go through daily. Please, PLEASE listen to what I'm telling the American girls out there. ACCEPT yourself for who you are and make self improvements based on what YOU want. Do not give up on yourself. It's not worth it. Do NOT let anyone tell you you're a bad person. It's not worth it. Do NOT let the media rule your mind and heart. It's not worth it. Do NOT let yourself go down too far. IT'S NOT WORTH IT.

Make yourself healthy, not just skinny. Looking in the mirror now, I'm still floored by what I've accomplished. Keep going, even when you feel it's harder to go on. Once you reach mini-goals, like five pounds gone, it gets easier. You will get stronger. You will get thinner. It takes time and it will happen for you. Just don't give up. Whatever you do, don't give up. The best feeling in the world is accomplishing something you have wanted for so long. The worst feeling is being so close to reaching a dream, then letting it slip away. Weight scales only measure earth's gravitational pull on your body, not your muscle-to-fat ratio or you as a person. Look in the mirror and FORGET THE SCALE.

This is probably the hardest task of them all. The scale gets imbedded in your mind and weight obsession kicks in. Letting the scale rule your life and own mind is ridiculous. If you don't like what's in the mirror, then change it. Don't let a stupid scale tell you what to do. You're the one in charge and you will always be. Muscle weighs three times more than fat (one pound of muscle=three pounds of fat). So if you're doing a lot of weight training, you're going to have more muscle mass than a thin person who doesn't do strength training, causing you to weigh some more. But you'll get leaner and stronger from the weights and burn more calories because muscle eats through more calories.

Most important of all, a scale definitely does not measure how much you have or have to accomplish. It will never measure you as a person. If you're satisfied with the person in the mirror, you're scale should only read

HAPPY. That's right. Put a sticky note with HAPPY ☺ on it if you have to. Well do it anyways, because it will make your day better. If you still want to improve some more, slap a note on the scale reader screen as IN PROGRESS. Or you could always just take a permanent black marker and black out the entire screen. It's ok. Do yourself a favor and just look at yourself once in the mirror a day to determine if you're actually happy with how you look.

Know what makes you happy and write it down right here right now.

My happy=:

1.
2.
3.
4.
5.
6.

7.

8.

9.

10.

If you can't fill all of the spaces in, that's perfectly fine. Find at least one object or activity, whether it's working out or gardening, that makes you happy. Whenever you're feeling like crap, pull the list out and do what's on the list, as long as it's healthy and legal.

Getting a happier mindset is a key to success in anything, not just getting healthy and weight loss. Even if it's just one thing, that one thing will help you stay focused and motivated! Also, picking a workout that makes you the happiest will help a ton. On your worst days, turning to that happy workout will make you feel so much better than if you had just sat on the couch. It's your go-to workout when you're in doubt or distress (or just want to do it over and over because you love it!).

Depression and even mild unhappiness can lead to eating problems, like eating too much or not enough. I went into a depression (my grandpa died of cancer) right before I started getting healthy, and I gained 12 pounds in only a month from overeating! Emotions can control your eating habits, so be aware of warning flags such as mindless eating or lack thereof at all times. No food is that good to where you have to look down at the scale and think, "Crap. This *really* sucks." I definitely know how that feels.

Staying positive can become hard when it takes longer to lose the weight. You get frustrated and maybe end up falling off the fitness wagon by skipping workouts or eating junk food. Don't obsess over setbacks! Obsessing over a slip or two (or even three or more) will take over your mindset! It will drive you absolutely nuts! Realize what you did wrong, fix it, and move on. Obsession over eating a couple french fries turns happy thinking into a complete self-bashing destruction for a lot of people. Feeling a little remorse and self-disappointment is expected, but weeks and months of mentally beating yourself up isn't. Yeah, I would freak out, too, if I had a major setback. But some people use the anger and frustration of setbacks as more fuel to their fitness fire, emerging stronger-willed than before. Know how you react to setbacks and know how to manage yourself based on your reactions. Just don't let setbacks throw you for the loop because you will regret it.

PART 4

THE LISTS

New workouts to try (high impact workouts are in bold):

—Biking/cycling (indoor/outdoor)

—Running

—Jogging

—Walking

—Swimming

—Weight lifting

—Resistance bands training

—Elliptical machine

—Cardio intervals

—Cardio/strength intervals

—Kickboxing/Karate

—Basketball

—Soccer

—Tennis

—Baseball

—Dancing (Latino/hip-hop/samba/pop)

—Jump roping

—Abs/core (crunches, trunk twists, weighted crunches, stability ball)

—Stability ball training

—Kettle ball training

—Hiking

—Kayaking

—Golfing

Note: You can always modify high-impact workouts and make low-impact workouts high impact. Impact means how much stress is being exerted on your joints and bones, not how intense the workout is. Low-impact workouts can have high-intensity.

Write down your favorite workouts here:

1.
2.
3.
4.
5.
6.
7.
8.
9.
10.

You can do a long workout of just one activity, or do a series of activities for shorter time spans each. Write down your favorite combinations here:

1.
2.
3.
4.
5.

Write down what time of the day you plan to work out each day here:

Sunday—
Monday—
Tuesday—
Wednesday—
Thursday—
Friday—
Saturday—

Writing down your workouts and at what time keeps you on track by keeping you organized! You also spend less time trying to figure out what work outs to do and spend more time getting things done! Staying organized is vital for everyone, but is especially crucial if you have a busy schedule.

Write down some favorite QHMs (quick healthy meals) here to fix on your busiest days:

1.

2.

3.

4.

5.

So busy you don't have time to cook? Order smart choices at fast-food chains such as salads (use your own dressing if fat-free options are unavailable), fruit, yogurt, and grilled meats (use your own wheat bun). Avoid anything fried!

Remember, you can do this! Never give up because of small or big obstacles! Stay on task, plan ahead, and be organized! If nothing else, keep your determination and motivation on high!

THE WORKOUT
TIPS

FORM OVER SPEED

CARDIO

When doing cardio, it's easy to get worn out and then get sloppy on form. Bad form doesn't really get you the workout you want. If your form starts to "fail" (sloppy), go slower instead of stopping, and get right back to where you were as fast as you can. Always jump from bent knees, never straight legs! Even though bending your knees takes an extra second or two, it will save your muscles and knees from wear and tear. You may not get as many jumps with bent knees than with straight knees in the interval, but protecting your knees and joints must be a priority. You don't want to have major knee or joint troubles in life at all if it can be helped. Taking the necessary precautions in your form, no matter how fast the cardio pace is, will help your body out in the long run.

STRENGTH/RESISTANCE BANDS

Form here is really crucial to prevent muscles from tearing or becoming overworked or stretched. If you're going at a faster pace (or more reps), go on the lighter side with the weights. If you're going at a slower pace (or fewer reps), you can lift heavier. But no matter fast or slow, keep good form and don't get sloppy! Keep your knees over your ankles when lifting weights or resistance bands! That means to not let your knees jut out over your ankles when doing exercises like squats. Jutting knees causes pain and issues where they should not be. With other resistance moves, pay attention to other people's form in the class or on the DVD. If you don't have either of those options, here's a quick list of basic form for some typical resistance moves.

Lateral shoulder lifts: The weights are in your palms. Keep elbows slightly bent and lift with your shoulders, not your neck. Hands and elbows should line up on the same plane.

Squats: Keep knees over ankles by sticking your butt back. Put the pressure on your heals (if you feel like you're falling backward, you're doing it right).

Bicep curls: Keep elbows at your hip, don't let them lift off or slide back or forward. Relax your grip so your forearms don't fatigue before your biceps.

Tricep kickbacks: Do one side at a time or both arms at once. Bend your knees and keep your elbow(s) above your back and in the same position (don't let them fall or slide around). If doing one arm at a time, keep the resting arm on your thigh.

Chest fly/press: Lay down on the floor or mat. Relax your grip. With flys, the weights go out to the sides; with presses, arms are at 90 degrees and go straight up. Don't strain your neck or let your elbows touch the floor too long. Don't go too heavy: the weight could fall on you!

MODIFY WHEN NEEDED

Not everyone is an Olympic athlete who can go all out every day with every workout. If you're doing a new workout, it's ok to modify the exercises until you know what you're doing or feel you can do the moves all out. Especially if you're new to working out in general, modify the moves until you build up your stamina to do the workouts unmodified. People with certain knee or joint issues need to modify certain workouts, too. Typical modifications are not jumping, lifting a lighter weight, or doing push-ups on your knees. Different workout DVDs or classes will usually show you the modifications for the moves. When in doubt, just go slower or lighter. On a workout machine like a treadmill or cycle, use less resistance or incline and go at a slower speed. Even top athletes need to modify moves when they get worn out towards the end of a workout. It's better to modify the moves in order to keep going than to stop or injure yourself.

PACE YOURSELF

Pacing yourself is key to any workout in order to complete it. Running and cardio are the workouts that typically get the most "pace yourself" advice, but strength trainers need to pace themselves as well. Pacing yourself is really important when running long distances or doing cardio for more than 30 minutes at a shot so you don't get a burn out early in the workout. Strength training needs pacing so you can maintain form and keep lifting throughout the workout. If you do more than you can handle early on, you'll run out of gas and burn out before you're done. If you're new to working out, this may sound a little foreign. Once you start working out, you'll know what your limits are and know how to pace yourself throughout various workouts. The pace for one cardio or strength workout may be different than the pace for a different one. There isn't any right or wrong pace to any workout because all workouts are highly individualized. Go at your own pace so you can maintain form and get through the whole workout. Over time, you'll get to where you can go faster, farther, and longer in various workouts, some in a shorter time than others.

PUSH YOURSELF

Pushing yourself is also really important in any workout. There isn't a formula to find the perfect balance between pacing and pushing in every kind of workout for everybody. An indicator that you can do more in a workout is if you don't feel worn out towards the end. Finish strong and do more right from the start the next time you do that workout. If you know you can lift ten pounds, lift ten, not five. Everyone is going to have a different starting point in workouts. Some people are able to go crazy and do high-energy workouts right away, others can't. That's ok! Know your personal fitness level in order to do the right workouts. If you're new to working out, try to lift five pounds when doing resistance training. For cardio, try to reach a level of 4 for you on a scale of 0-10 (0=resting, 10=hardest you can go). This scale is different for everyone with every workout. You might be able to run faster than you can punch in kickboxing or lift heavier on one type of squat versus another kind. Do the most you can the first time around and try to do more the next time you go through that workout. Don't give up and finish strong no matter what workout you're doing! Work up to that all-out level by doing a little more each time!

BUILD UP TO HEAVIER WEIGHTS

If you're not sure how heavy to lift, stick with five pounds for everything. Starting out, I could barely pick up a five pound weight, so that was a good weight to start with. If five pounds feels too light or easy, try eight or ten pounds. If your form gets sloppy, go down to a lighter weight until you can lift the heavier weight. Different muscle groups gain strength at different rates for everyone. Your legs may be able to handle more weight in a faster amount of time than say your shoulders. Bigger muscle groups like the legs and back typically can lift more weight than smaller groups like triceps and posterior deltoids (the back of the shoulder). Biceps, chest, and the medial deltoids (the main shoulder muscle in the middle) are usually somewhere in between the larger and smaller muscle groups for most people. When the weight you're lifting feels too light, increase your weight by five pounds, but no more than ten. You don't want to go from five to twenty pounds overnight because your muscles will tear and you won't be able to work out. A little soreness for a day or two is normal and a good sign because that means the muscles are changing. However, extreme pain or limpness for several days isn't-go to a doctor to make sure the muscles are not torn. Hot showers and over the counter pain meds help out with typical muscle soreness.

WORK OUT AROUND MINOR INJURIES

Muscle soreness and other minor workout miffs are irritating, but they go away within a couple days. Avoid the muscle groups that are sore for a couple days, but don't not workout. Cardio helps work muscle soreness out. If you're doing strength training the next workout and your legs are sore, just avoid doing squats and other leg moves; focus instead on your upper body. Broken bones are usually the death sentence for workout fanatics, but don't let it be! If your leg is broken, you can still work out your upper body with punches and upper body moves (vice versa for an upper body injury). However, if you're in excruciating pain or have a major injury, don't attempt to workout. Ask your doctor for specifics and to confirm how serious the injury is. When I got my wisdom teeth removed, I asked the doctor when I could work out again. He said whenever I felt ok; I worked out the next morning because I fortunately had no complications and felt perfectly fine. However, know your own body. Get plenty of rest so when you're fully recovered, you'll be ready to get back into the workout routine. Depending on how long your recovery time is, you may need to go easy the first few days back working out until you get the hang of it again and don't reinjure yourself. Play injuries by ear and always check with a doctor to make sure you're ok to get back in the game.

GO EASIER WHEN SICK

Obviously, if you're puking you're guts out with the flu, you're not going to work out, so don't even try because it'll get ugly. Instead, wait it out and gradually build up your workouts after you get better. Keep eating healthy when you can keep food and liquids down. Healthy food will help you recover faster and better after being really sick than treating yourself to junk food because junk food does nothing to help your body get over an illness.

When the typical but irritating cold arises, it's not an alarm to stop working out altogether. Even the top athletes get the sniffles in the winter or during allergy season. Just make your workouts a little easier so your symptoms don't worsen. Mild headaches and sinus congestion prove to be a nuisance when working out, but working out at an easier pace usually helps and gets your mind off of it. However, major headaches like migraines and severe congestion in the form of bronchitis means a day or two without working out (or working out at a much easier or slower pace). Everyone has a different threshold for illness, so like injuries, play illnesses by ear. If you feel up to working out at your normal or a moderate pace, go for it, but be aware that it may worsen your symptoms. Severe illnesses could create a workout setback, depending on the nature of the illness, but your body will need to rest and recover, so listen to your doctor about how serious your illness is.

PAY ATTENTION

Safety has to be the top priority in any workout, no matter what or where it is. An obvious example is paying extra special attention to your surroundings when working out outside, such as running or biking. You should never ever workout in any area where there are few to no streetlights or is away from public facilities. This is a safety precaution that could mean life or death in the most extreme cases. If possible, work out with a buddy or a group if you're running or biking between cities or at night. Always have a cell phone on hand and wear bright colored clothes. Have a backup plan in case of a storm, malfunction, or other obstacle. Never go out on open water to swim, kayak, or the like in the middle of a storm or on the brink of one.

Less obvious safety hazards involve equipment and weights. If you don't know how to operate a specific work out machine, ask someone who does know so you don't get hurt. Never lift more weight than you feel capable of to prevent dropping weights on your face or feet and to prevent hurting your back. Don't wear any dangling jewelry or shoe laces when using cardio or weight equipment because they could get caught in the machine. With any workout, make sure you have enough room around to do it so you don't get hurt. Nothing hurts worse than doing a back kick straight into the glass coffee table or jumping up right into the ceiling. So be cautious when you work out, so you can work out every day safely.

KNOW PERSONAL WORK OUT DETAILS

Knowing basic little details like how you like to work out will help you stay motivated and keep you on track. If you get distracted when working out with someone else, then work out by yourself to get things done. Others find that working out with one or more other people keeps them going in their workouts and challenges them to go harder. A lot of people love to work out to music. I can't work out without having heart-pumping music blasting in the background! Music keeps you going and pushes you to go the extra mile. Certain fast-paced songs will make you do more than you would not have done otherwise.

Find out what time of the day you like to work out. Some people need to work out first thing in the morning because they know that during the day they're crunched for time. Others want to work out late at night, still others like to work out sometime during the day. If you loathe getting up early or staying up really late, then avoid the times you hate during the day. If you work out at a time when you're uncomfortable, chances are you'll associate that unlikable time with working out and not want to work out. So know yourself and your schedule. Make time to work out how you want-it will be the best thing you will do for yourself!

BE PATIENT

Ok, so this tip is really, really hard to follow. It's probably the hardest one of them all. I'm extremely impatient; I want things to get done as fast as possible, including getting results from working out. When you're trying to lose weight or just get in better shape, time slows to a snail crawl. It seems as though it's still day one of a new workout routine, even when it's several weeks into it. You can see the end of the road, but getting there feels as though it'll take eons. When I first started out, I planned on it taking two years to lose fifty pounds—it only took the majority of a school year! For some people, losing weight or getting in shape will take a long time, depending on much weight you want to lose or your fitness goals. The old phrase "Rome wasn't built in a day" definitely applies here. It will take several months at least to see a moderate difference in your appearance and/or weight. But every day, your body is getting stronger and fitter, maybe even losing a fraction of a pound a day in some cases, whether the mirror and scale shows it. On day one, you could barely do a push-up at all. On day five, maybe you can do two or three. Within two or three weeks, maybe you can crank out a solid set of twelve or more. The point is, you got to stick with the program. Don't expect to see results overnight because that's not how it works. Don't give up after a couple days of frustration-you will get better in your workouts! If you don't reach your exact goals on an exact day, it's ok! Just keep on going no matter what and you will be glad you did. I know it gets hard to be patient and wait. I thought the final pounds would never come off, but they did, and I've never regretted not giving up and staying on task. I don't want you to set unrealistic expectations, because you won't reach them and you'll get extremely disappointed and probably will quit. Set realistic goals based on what you want to achieve or how much weight you want to lose, stick to it, and be patient, and you will get there. Hang in there and it will happen for you.

The Start of a New Beginning

Papaw—

When I was born, you quit smoking. When you died, I began my new healthier lifestyle. You fought stage 4 cancer for eight and a half years. I struggled with my weight being the fat kid for eight and a half years. In 2008, cancer ended your life too soon. In 2008, I found my new beginning and what I was missing for so long in my life. Thank you for showing me how to put up a relentless fight to get the most out of life and to overcome a combat with your health. I've realized that this wasn't just the end of something . . . it was a whole new beginning. Not just a whole new size, but also a whole new life. You have to have the inner willpower and strength to carry on, to keep going, to keep the fire ignited to not just survive but also to thrive. You showed me how to not give up on yourself, no matter what the doctors say, by having a wildfire need to keep on living the best you can. I've never regretted giving all I can towards being the healthiest I can be, and I will never end this fight. The torch of willpower to live the healthiest I can has been ignited and will never be put out. Thank you for showing me how to give it all that you got no matter what happens.

So now, to those reading the end of this book, don't let anything make you give up on yourself. Your life should be lived the healthiest it can be because you only get one body and one life. Your life will be so much better when you take care of yourself, not just to be thin and in shape. It should not just be a battle of the bulge in the mirror, but also a war against anything that threatens your well being, your health, your personal goals and happiness. This is so much more than the end of bad habits and frustration—this is the beginning of a new you, a new life. So go get it with all that you got. You'll never regret it.

THANK YOU

A huge shout-out to the woman that ignited my love of working out, kickboxing in particular: Chalene Johnson! I cannot possibly thank you enough for creating the most amazing workouts I've ever done! I remember the first day I tried one of your kickboxing workouts. It was a humid and hot day in August 2008, and this was around the time that I realized that I needed to change my unhealthy lifestyle. There was this little cardboard box in my house with some dust on it, filled with the set of "TurboJam" DVDs. I had already attempted to work out on the elliptical at home, but without any vigor. I fingered through the little booklet that came with it and figured on trying the workouts. I popped the 15-minute one in and five minutes into it, an amazing thing happened. I absolutely loved it! I had never in my life loved working out that much. It was unbelievable! Then I did the 20-minute one, too, and I worked out the very next day with those DVDs. My working out was delayed by a couple weeks because of having a minor foot procedure done, but then I got right back into it. In October, I got really serious about what I ate, completely cutting out the super-high calorie crap I was eating and foregoing my bowl of cereal or ice cream right before bed. By the end of November, I had lost nearly 15 pounds! I kept going and going, getting stronger every week and pushing myself to kick harder and jump higher. I never thought I would lose five pounds, much less 50. I combined the kickboxing with some heavier weights in the spring, but during the winter I did some different workouts to mix things up so I didn't hit a plateau. Thank you for your energy, for your passion for fitness, for your groundbreaking workouts . . . I know I would not be where I am today if it wasn't for you. Thank you so much for being the wonderful role model and fitness fanatic that you are. You have inspired me to live life to the fullest in the healthiest way possible and have inspired millions to do the same.

I'm currently a high school student who loves fitness and health. I gained a lot of weight from the age of 7 and was humiliated all the time because I was always the fat girl in school. In eighth grade, I took it upon myself to lose the weight (50 pounds) for reasons besides avoiding the embarrassment of being a fat kid. My grandpa died of cancer a few months before then, so that was a huge wake up call that life is short and to live it like it should be lived in a healthy way. Another wake up call was later that year in the summer. I was watching a show on T.V. about obese kids going to hospitals to get weight loss surgery. A teenage boy on the show suffocated because of his own body weight and died in the hospital. The lethal combination of teasing, embarrassment, and looming death proved the fuel to my motivational fire. I was sick of being teased, tired of wearing women's clothes, and fed up with being the fat girl. I have not eaten any junk food, sweets, or soda for over three years now. And I mean NOT ONE BITE (or even a lick). I still consistently work out every day for two hours, from kickboxing to dancing to weight lifting to cycling. I know how it is to feel to be the fat kid and how hard the going gets from the embarrassment and teasing, something so many top-notch doctors and weight loss specialists can't vouch for. My other extreme loves are my love of animals and music. I adore animals, especially fuzzy and marine ones. I have two yellow Labs, an adopted Shih-Tzu, and an adopted chocolate lop-eared bunny (and a fish tank). I don't know what I would do without my fuzzy cuties-they're always there for me! I'm addicted to pop and hip-hop music and am always envisioning music video concepts for songs. I love Lady Gaga's music; she's my absolute favorite! I also love the music of Beyonce, Katy Perry, Nick Minaj, Rhianna, Pink, and Britney Spears. My entire life and heart revolves around health and fitness, animals, and music; those are the three greatest things in the world for me! I live in Poquoson, Virginia. It's a small seafood town where everyone knows everybody and is a really great little city; it's where I've lived my whole life!